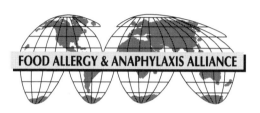

FOOD ALLERGY & ANAPHYLAXIS ALLIANCE

Stories from the Heart

A Collection of Essays From Teens
with Food Allergies

Volume II

Table of Contents

Table of Contents (continued)

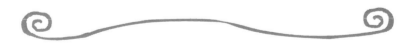

Introduction

When the first volume of this series was published, we received numerous letters thanking us for finally presenting the opportunity for teens to share their food allergy experiences. The response was so tremendous that we couldn't resist publishing a second volume.

The teen years are full of exciting, frustrating, and emotional experiences. There are times it feels like there is no one else going through the same experiences or emotions. We hope that in reading these stories, you'll realize that there are many teens who are right there beside you—whether you are trying to explain your allergy to your friends and classmates, coping with how to handle a reaction, or just learning as you go along.

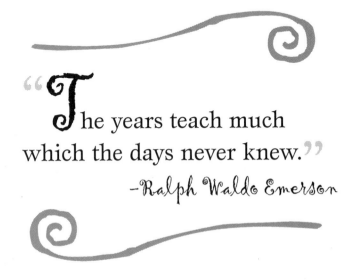

"The years teach much which the days never knew."

—Ralph Waldo Emerson

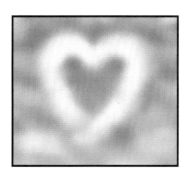

Part One: Life's Lessons

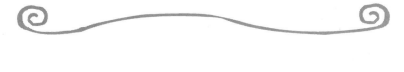

"The people who get on in this world are the people who get up and look for the circumstances they want, and if they can't find them, make them."

—George Bernard Shaw

An Open Letter to My Allergens

Dear Dairy Products, Peanuts, Eggs, and Seafood,

I'm sorry, but I just can't eat you. Don't take it personally, I have nothing against you. When I eat you I get sick. You know—I can't breathe, I get a horrible stomachache, I vomit, I break out in hives and rashes, my mouth itches, and I don't feel like myself for days afterward. I've been avoiding you for most of my life, but now, after a year of college, some things need to be said between us.

Ever since I can remember, I have been vigilantly on the lookout for you, making sure I never eat anything that contains you as ingredients. I used to always wear a bracelet with a message inscribed telling people not to feed you to me. I learned which foods were safe for me and which foods were not. Almost as soon as I could read, I was checking the ingredient labels on foods for myself.

In fourth grade, I went to a weeklong overnight camp for the first time. They weren't prepared for the extensive range of my allergies. All I could eat the whole week was fruit, oatmeal, and chicken. I had to talk to the cook about the meals and helped her find recipes I could eat. I learned a lot about myself that week and about my ability to communicate with others to take care of myself. I

Kathryn,
age 19
Allergic to milk,
peanuts, eggs,
and fish
USA

5

bring the sense of responsibility from monitoring my diet from a young age into other aspects of my life, be it schoolwork, my job, or my encounters and relationships with other people.

Other people have helped me all my life in dealing with you. Allergists and doctors have diagnosed and treated my allergies. My parents made adjustments and found creative solutions to the challenges posed by my food allergies. My first-grade teacher kept licorice in her desk so that I would have something to eat when my classmates brought in birthday treats.

Benevolent wait staff in restaurants have dug through the kitchen to find ingredient statements. Friends and relatives help watch out for me and often go out of their way to make sure I have something to eat. They have all showed me the importance of helping others and being aware of their needs.

I feel that I owe the same compassion to members of my community and the rest of the world. Working with children is an important way for me to better others' lives.

Recently, I volunteered as a camp counselor, and my experiences with my food allergies made it easier for me to relate to the children. There were two little girls in my group who were also allergic to you. The three of us had a special relationship as we all ate meals without you in them together. Being allergic to you helps me relate to others because I know that everyone has their own obstacles and struggles. With each passing day I find myself growing more and more capable of giving back the same compassion that I have been shown.

Our relationship doesn't adhere to the prevailing norms of society. I have gained a more sensitive perception of the world and what is currently occurring around me from my experiences with you. I am very conscious of how lucky I am to have the ability to receive the medical attention I need. This awareness of the fragility of life helps me to appreciate everything more. I am also more determined to live life to its fullest.

Avoiding you is a formidable and burdensome challenge. You have been the source of many trials and traumas. However, I realize that I would never, ever have become who I am now without you. My whole realm of experiences would be different. You do not define me, but my attitude and response to the challenges you pose are reflective of my character. I approach the obstacles you create with a positive, productive attitude that helps me to learn and grow from my experiences with you.

Sincerely,

Kathryn

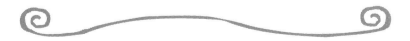

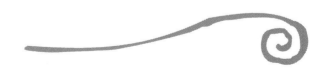

"Friends are angels who lift us to our feet when our wings have trouble remembering how to fly."

—Anonymous

If I knew then what I know now, life would be different. If I knew then what I know now, then I might not have eaten that ice cream with nuts on it. Unfortunately, I did not know anything about food allergies when I had my first reaction.

If I knew when I was only 8 years old that eating certain foods could be fatal, surely I would have been better off. I would have avoided ingesting foods that triggered reactions. I had never heard of anaphylactic shock, and I definitely never thought that something like that could happen to me.

In fact, the first utterance I heard of those two words (anaphylactic shock) was when I was lying in the intensive care unit because of what I had eaten. If I knew how to use the EpiPen,® then maybe I could have prevented my reactions from progressing. If only I had known to read the ingredient statements on food packages before eating the food in them. All of these ifs!

If only life were that easy and you knew all of the hardships that were to come. It is too bad that we have no idea what we may encounter in the coming months. But there can also be good aspects of not knowing what will happen. The element of surprise can be good.

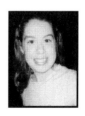

Kari,
age 13
Allergic to peanuts
and tree nuts
USA

If my food allergies could have been prevented, I would not be greeted with all of the assistance that I get wherever I go. I might miss the special attention that I get. You can learn a lot from your past experiences, regardless of whether they are positive or negative.

If I had known before one of my reactions that I was allergic to a specific food, then I would have stayed away from it. I would never have known what it was like to go through a reaction or have a near-death experience. Consequently, I would have spent my whole life wondering what would happen to me if I ate peanut butter. But I would never have taken the chance with my life that I unknowingly took when I ate the things I am allergic to.

There is a saying about life: live and learn. If I knew then what I know now about what can result from eating certain foods, then my life would definitely be different, in both positive and negative ways. I could have prevented my experiences, but then I would not have known what could possibly happen. I feel that I am in the best possible situation right now, knowing what to expect from a reaction and also having enough knowledge to try to prevent one.

I am thankful that I know now what I did not know then.

My advice to others...

Always read ingredient statements! Don't let your food allergies stop you from doing what you want.

About Kari...

Siblings: One sister, Jackie, age 12

Career goals: Teacher

Hobbies/interests: Ballet, playing the clarinet, using AOL, and reading

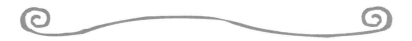

"It is good to have an end to journey toward; but it is the journey that matters, in the end."

— Ursula K. Le Guin

The Positive Side of an Allergy

I am 17 and will be heading off to college soon. My allergy declared its presence when I was 2. I was sitting in a small room when a vacuum-packed jar of peanuts was opened. My face and lips began to swell grotesquely. Subsequent allergy testing revealed my extreme sensitivity to peanuts.

My parents and I are not big risk takers when it comes to keeping me alive, so we have adhered to a strict and very simple rule: I never eat a single bite of food unless it is prepared under the watchful eye of my parents or myself. This has definitely been a cumbersome policy, but it has paid off in comfort and safety, as I have never once experienced a reaction to peanuts since the day I was diagnosed.

It has been a nuisance to plan every bite of food in advance; it has destroyed many opportunities for a spontaneous meal with my friends. While I have suffered some in this regard, the importance of thinking before I act has become deeply ingrained within me. I differ from those of my peers who do anything they choose on a whim, without giving any thought to possible consequences.

We all know that there is a major downside to having a severe food allergy. The amazing discovery I have made is that there is a positive side to having such an allergy as well.

I have done quite a bit of traveling over the years because I am a serious

Patrick,
age 17
Allergic to peanuts
USA

competitive chess player. I always bring my own meals with me when I travel, especially to international competitions, but there have been some benefits. I have savored many delicious homemade meals on airplanes while those around me have suffered through awful airplane food.

At high-level international chess tournaments, any given match may extend late into the night. While having to travel with my own food has been a hassle, it has been nice to have a prepared meal waiting in my cooler upon returning from a long match at a late hour. I would have enjoyed eating with my peers at a restaurant, but I was just as happy to have been able to eat quickly and get to sleep.

Even in common social settings, it is sometimes nice to be able to eat my own food. Since people I visit know that I strictly adhere to a policy of eating only food I have brought for myself, I have been able to gracefully duck out of eating some pretty nasty stuff!

I am moving out of state for college, so I will need to cook for myself from the day I arrive at school. The housing department at my college is providing me with an on-campus apartment to help meet my needs. So that I can drive to the grocery store, I have been granted an exemption from the ban on freshman having cars on campus. Those are two pretty nice perks that I will be enjoying because of my allergy.

My extreme allergy to peanuts has significantly impacted my lifestyle in both positive and negative ways. Given the choice, I would prefer to have been born without it. However, the fact is that it also has some beneficial effects on my life and has been a much more tolerable condition than one might imagine.

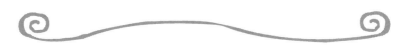

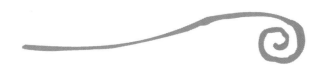

"There are many ways of going forward, but only one way of standing still."

—Franklin D. Roosevelt

There have been many times in my life when things have gone wrong with my milk allergy. However, from all these experiences with others, I have learned a lot, and I feel that if I share my experiences with others, they will be able to avoid "accidents" in the future. Here are the top five lessons that I have learned in my 17 years.

First, I would have avoided sitting next to little boys who took great pleasure in flicking their straws out of their milk cartons. When I was in preschool, a boy I was sitting next to during lunch did just that. The milk from the straw landed in my eye, causing it to swell so much that it appeared to be turning inside out. Today, I still have to be careful, because those little boys grow up and then start throwing larger items, such as pizza.

Next, I would have been more careful about which mashed potatoes I was eating. My mom would always make separate mashed potatoes for me, but one time, I guess she was in too much of a hurry and gave me the wrong potatoes. Today, since I am old enough, I pretty much take care of my own food, which works out fine. My advice to parents is that maybe they should try to put food coloring in the potatoes. Plus, they could get festive with it. Red and green for Christmas?

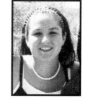

Jessica,
age17
Allergic to milk
USA

Third, I would have never taken the risk of eating out at a restaurant. These days, people are just not aware of how severe an allergy can be. Although you may tell your server that you have an allergy to a certain food, there is no guarantee that your food will be safe. Why take the risk? Instead, order a drink and enjoy the company you are with. Even though you don't get to eat, I promise you that not eating is a lot more enjoyable than spending the night in the hospital.

Fourth, I would have always made sure that any kitchen utensil that I used was thoroughly cleaned. Once, when I was little, my aunt cut my hamburger with a knife that had been previously used to cut a cheeseburger. Although I only had a small reaction, I did not enjoy being sick when all of my cousins were running around playing. My advice is that you should always make sure all dishes and utensils are clean before using them. Also, if you are allergic to milk, like me, distinctive cups are also highly recommended.

Finally, in all seriousness, I would use my EpiPen® immediately upon ingesting any food that had milk in it. If you wait, it could cost you more than you bargained for. I carry my EpiPen® with me at all times, even when I don't think I will need it.

I have had many experiences that have helped me learn how to deal better with my anaphylaxis to milk. I hope that I can help others learn how to cope with their allergies and avoid some of the "accidents" that I have had.

My advice to others...

Allergies shouldn't stop you from doing what you want to do. Just plan ahead.

About Jessica...

Siblings: One brother, Joey, age 15; one stepbrother, Corey, age 16

Career goals: Teacher or interior designer

Hobbies/interests: Reading, hiking, camping, hanging out with friends, and watching movies

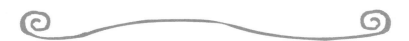

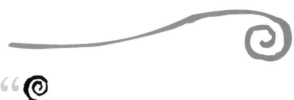

"Experience is the one thing you can't get for nothing."

–Oscar Wilde

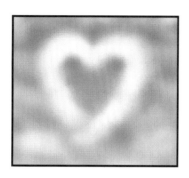

Part Two: Allergic Reactions

"*Patience and perseverance have a magical affect before which difficulties disappear and obstacles vanish.*"

—John Quincy Adams

*N*ovember 27, 1996, was a day that opened my eyes. Before then, I never realized how serious my food allergies were. I also never realized the importance of each and every day I walk this earth. That was because November 27, 1996, was nearly the last day of my life.

My parents first discovered my allergy to walnuts when I was 11 months old. I had touched an unopened bag of walnuts, causing my arms to break out in hives. As it turned out, I was also allergic to peanuts and many other tree nuts.

November 27, 1996, was the day before Thanksgiving. As a high school sophomore, I was celebrating the coming holiday with my homeroom class. There were many cookies brought by students for the party. I knew there were some cookies on the table that I dare not eat.

I knew this when I bit into a cookie that looked safe that November morning. I also knew what happened when I ate a food containing nuts—I felt sick. What I didn't know was how dangerous taking a chance with my food allergies could be.

Andy,
age 20
Allergic to peanuts
and tree nuts
USA

It wasn't until I had eaten the entire cookie that my throat began to swell up. When I discovered that the cookie contained walnuts, I called home. My mom picked me up and brought me to our house, where I threw up just like I had every other time I had ingested nuts.

This time, however, something was different. Never before had I suddenly found myself gasping for breath. When my breathing didn't improve, my mom and I decided she should give me my epinephrine injection and drive me to the hospital. We hadn't even gotten a mile before I passed out and stopped breathing.

The next thing I remember was finding myself in the emergency room. There were nurses all around me. I couldn't speak because I had a tube down my throat. Luckily my mom, dad, and grandparents were all standing by, all very happy to see that I had regained consciousness.

Although there is much I don't remember, the story of what happened that day will stay in my mind forever. I had gone into anaphylactic shock and nearly died.

It took the help of many doctors, nurses, technicians, and paramedics to keep my heart beating. And that wasn't everyone who helped me. As I was later told, my mom had to dodge traffic on slippery roads in her race to the hospital. At one intersection, when she was finally stuck, a couple rushed to our aid by directing traffic, following our car, and carrying me into the hospital. Weeks later, we were able to contact the couple and thank them for their help. They even made it to my graduation party three years later, which meant a lot to me.

That Thanksgiving was a very emotional one. After I recuperated in the ICU, my parents and I made the trip back home. I had never been so happy to see my family as I was that night for Thanksgiving dinner. We all had so much to be thankful for—my mom's bravery, the couple that helped her in traffic, and all the medical miracle-workers who kept me alive.

Since that day, I've never forgotten how lucky I am to be alive. I remember this each and every day. I also remember how serious my food allergies are, and how important it is that I practice strict avoidance of nuts. In the four and a half years since the incident, I haven't had a single allergic reaction. Nonetheless, I always carry two epinephrine shots and wear a Medic Alert® necklace.

As much as my experience with anaphylaxis has changed my life, I would like to think it has also changed the lives of those around me. My parents and I have shared the story of my experience with countless others. After much research, my mom compiled a paper about the severity of nut allergies and how important it is for those with the allergies to avoid anything containing nuts. Her efforts have gained the attention of local news media, becoming part of the dramatic increase in publicity about nut allergies nationwide.

Thanks to my mom and many concerned individuals like her, the world now takes nut allergies much more seriously. Warnings are placed on products that may contain peanuts, and many airlines restrict the distribution of peanuts when an allergic individual is on board.

Because of my own incident, my high school trained its faculty and staff on what to do when a student has an allergic reaction and how to give an epinephrine injection. Due to a change in policy, the school must now call an ambulance immediately whenever a student ingests an allergen. The school has followed this protocol more than once.

I strongly believe that one day scientists will find a way to prevent reactions like mine from ever threatening another life. Until then, I will continue to count my blessings and do my part to keep the world around me informed about the many threats of food allergies.

My advice to others...

Never be afraid to ask questions about what's in food. Never take chances—play it safe.

About Andy...

Siblings: None

Career goals: Journalist

Hobbies/interests: Computers and improvisational comedy

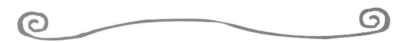

If You Can't Read It, Don't Eat It

My parents found out I had a peanut allergy when I was 8 months old. When my grandma gave me a bit of her peanut butter and jelly sandwich, I swelled everywhere and got hives. My parents were given epinephrine and instructions on how to keep me safe. I didn't have any more exposures until I was 5.

At a deli where I had eaten many times, I was given a cookie that I thought I had eaten before, but the server this time didn't know that it was a peanut butter cookie, not a chocolate chip one. I vomited immediately, my lips swelled, and I got hives all over my body. My mom knew this was the real thing, and she had an EpiPen® with us. We happened to be with a friend who was a nurse, who gave me the injection and then gave me Benadryl.® But instead of calling 911, the friend drove us to a hospital.

In the car on the way, I felt my airway closing. It was very scary. We got to the emergency room and they immediately gave me oxygen and medications. My mom was told I was in severe anaphylactic shock and that they would have to transport me to another hospital if I didn't pull out of it. Luckily I did, but I still had to spend the night in the ICU. Now I know what it feels like to have an anaphylactic reaction.

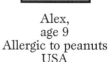

Alex,
age 9
Allergic to peanuts
USA

I am very careful about what I eat, even if it means I can't have what everyone else is eating. Our new rules are:

- If you can't read it, don't eat it.

- Always call 911; don't take yourself to the hospital.

- Carry at least two EpiPen®s.

I wish I didn't have this allergy, but my parents are pretty good about letting me do what other kids do. I go to school and eat lunch in the lunchroom, play sports, go to science camps, and am a Cub Scout. I just always have to have my EpiPen®s wherever I go.

My advice to others...

Always read the label. If you can't read it, don't eat it.

About Alex...

Siblings: Two sisters, Anna, age 7, and Michelle, age 3

Career goals: Aeronautical engineering or scientific research

Hobbies/interests: Collecting sports cards, playing computer games, and reading

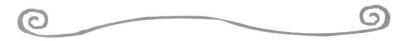

I was a bright, fidgety girl in third grade. On Valentine's Day that year I could have entirely cared less about icky love stuff and was instead enjoying my cupcake and some movie about sharks my teacher had put in.

A girl came up to me with a plate of cookies. I took a quick look. "Do they have any nuts in them?" I asked her. "No," she said, gaping at me like a goldfish. Well, I had asked like my mom told me to, so why not? I took a cookie and took a bite while I looked at the shark gliding along on the TV screen.

My throat suddenly got so dry I could barely swallow. I got up and took a drink of water and sat back down. I ended up doing this three more times, every time getting more nervous. I realized what I had done and walked up to my teacher. "I think I ate nuts," I squeaked, trying to swallow and not succeeding. She gave me one look and sent the student teacher down to the nurse with me.

We were silent as we walked as quickly as possible through the hallways to the little office full of big-eyed children trying to fake being sick. I don't remember what the student teacher told the nurse, but the next thing I knew she was putting on latex gloves and rummaging in her cabinet for my EpiPen.® She called Cookie Girl's mother and found out crushed walnuts were part of the recipe. "We're going to have

Ashley,
age 15
Allergic to peanuts
and tree nuts
USA

29

to give you a shot, Ashley," she said reluctantly. No kids were in the office now.

My reason and stability snapped. "No!" I freaked out, and began to jabber. "Give me Benadryl!® My mommy gave it to me when I had a reaction before!" I yelled over and over again, with the nurse frowning even harder. She would have taken my arm, but I ran away. She tried to catch me as I ran around the room in circles, still jabbering and hysterical. She gave up and called the front office.

The principal and vice principal walked in to find me crying and oppositional, with the poor nurse not knowing what to do. They got me to lie down on a cushioned bench, but I was not cooperating at all on my little adrenaline rush. I told the principal to go away in what seemed like the rudest way possible. "I will, but only if you calm down," she told me. Since nothing seemed worse than the indignity of taking a shot in front of the woman who controlled the school, not to mention that I could hardly breathe, I gave in, and the principal and vice principal left that part of the office.

They called an ambulance, rolled me out in a stretcher like I had broken my neck, and wouldn't let me sit up even though I felt fine. I met my agitated mother at the hospital.

"I thought she meant peanuts!" protested Cookie Girl afterward. I now understand the incredible risk I take when I eat something I have not cooked myself. Who would take a 9-year-old's word on something so complicated? Only someone who didn't understand the risk.

My advice to others...

It's not worth it to eat an allergen and have to deal with the misery. Always check labels with an eagle eye.

About Ashley...

Siblings: One sister, Allison, age 18

Career goals: Science field like genetics or epidemiology, or writer

Hobbies/interests: Playing field hockey, running, playing the violin, reading, sleeping, and computers

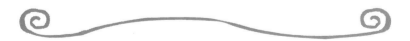

"*I* have learned from experience that the greater part of our happiness or misery depends on our dispositions and not on our circumstances."

—Martha Washington

*I*t all began when we went to pick up my dad from the airport on Friday night. I hugged my dad and said hi. On our way to dinner, I felt some of the symptoms of an allergic reaction to peanuts. My dad said he had eaten peanuts on the plane. I had a panic attack. My mom said we had to go to the hospital. Luckily, we were really close. With tears streaming down my scared face, we went to the emergency room.

My mom told the nurse what had happened and all the symptoms I had. We went into one of the rooms and in rushed the doctor. I told him what was going on and how I felt. The nurse put this bracelet on me. I was so nervous about what could happen to me. They had all the things they needed to give me an EpiPen® shot. The doctor told me I had to stay in the emergency room for at least an hour so he could keep a close eye on me to see if I needed the EpiPen.® I really didn't want to have to use the EpiPen,® but I knew it would be worth it.

Luckily, they didn't have to give me a shot but gave me Benadryl,® which is medicine that I hate and that makes me tired. I have to take it when I have an allergic reaction.

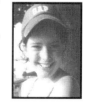

The doctor came in and asked how I was, and I said I felt a little better. About an hour later my dad and my sister, Hallie, came back with food. I was starved; no wonder I

Jacqueline,
age 11
Allergic to peanuts
USA

had a stomachache. In the hospital bed I had a Coke® and some fries. The fries weren't that warm, but it was the best I could have at the time. I was in the emergency room for about an hour, and I can tell you the emergency room is probably the scariest room you will ever be in. That is my life with a severe allergy to peanuts.

My advice to others...

If someone has a birthday and brings in treats at school, you don't always have to eat it. And remember, you are not the only kid that has to go through not eating whatever you want.

About Jacqueline...

Siblings: One sister, Hallie, age 8

Career goals: Professional tennis player

Hobbies/interests: Playing tennis, reading, writing, and hanging out with friends

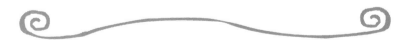

When I was about 2 years old, it was determined that I am deathly allergic to tree nuts. After that diagnosis, I was frequently taught about what course of action I was to take if I ever had a reaction. I knew to call 911 and use my EpiPen® immediately. I've also worn my Medic Alert® bracelet faithfully since I was 3. I had gone until my 12th summer without ever experiencing a reaction that could result in death.

One evening in August my mom brought home a box of oatmeal raisin cookies from a party. The box listed the ingredients, and my mom specifically told me she had read them and they did not include nuts. I asked if I could have one, but she replied, "No, not before dinner." However, when her head was turned, I read the ingredients as I had been trained to, grabbed a cookie, and ate it in one bite.

The instant the cookie was in my mouth, my throat closed. I had this terrible scratchy sensation as I slowly took deep breaths. I knew immediately something was terribly wrong; however, I was confused because the ingredient list stated the cookies did not contain nuts. Simultaneously, my mom and sister were preparing to go rent a movie, which would leave me with my dad. I followed them out to the car, still saying nothing because I felt guilty about disobeying my mother, and even more guilty that my defiance might lead to my first life-threatening reaction.

Michelle,
age 16
Allergic to peanuts
and tree nuts
USA

I had tears in my eyes as I watched them pull out of the driveway. Then I hurried inside and took an EpiPen® off my desk. At this time it had been about five minutes since I had eaten the cookie. I itched mercilessly, and my skin was swollen and flaming red. My lips bulged with hives, and my eyes were mere slits from the swelling. Finally, I climbed upstairs to my dad and told him what I'd done. I was absolutely petrified.

My breath came in short gasps, and I knew I could not make it much longer. I started repeating hysterically, "Oh please, Dad, help me, please..." He tried to get me down the stairs. I fell most of the way. He ran for the phone in the kitchen to call an ambulance, and I summoned the energy to give myself the epinephrine. With the shot given, I passed out in the kitchen. I vaguely remember staggering with my dad's support to the front porch. I was unconscious until the paramedics came.

In hindsight, I view this as a dramatic learning experience. The package had been mislabeled and contained walnuts. The entire episode took place within 10 to 15 minutes.

I have never again withheld the fact that I am having a reaction. During this first incident I was scared and naïve. Now, I am calm and efficient in handling my reactions. In a more recent reaction, I was able to call 911 at once and promptly use the EpiPen.® I am exceedingly cautious now; however, I have come to realize that accidents do happen.

When they do occur, I am confident that I can follow through with the steps to save my life.

My advice to others...

I consider my allergies a unique part of who I am. It's one of the best conversation starters I've found. Also, enlist the help of your friends. The support and fascination I have come across concerning my allergies is amazing.

About Michelle...

Siblings: One sister, Mary, age 14

Career goals: Ambassador to the United Nations

Hobbies/interests: Competitive swimming, playing water polo, singing, and coaching younger kids

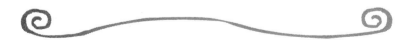

"A happy person is not a person in a certain set of circumstances, but rather a person with a certain set of attitudes."

—Hugh Downs

One afternoon at 3:30, after school, I had one of the worst days of my life. I was 10 years old. It was just a few days before Easter that I experienced this horrible moment.

The bell rang and I was very excited because my hockey try-outs were after school. My friend Kyle had won a big basket full of chocolate. About halfway between my house and the school, Kyle asked me if I wanted a chocolate egg. I asked him, "What kind of chocolate is it?" He said, "It's a mini Kinder Surprise®". Usually, regular-sized Kinder Surprise®s have no peanuts or any other type of nuts inside. So I thought that it was going to be the same thing. But, boy, was I ever wrong.

I opened the wrapping paper of the chocolate. There were no ingredients in or on the outside of it. But, since it was a Kinder Surprise,® I figured that I would be okay. I took the chocolate and put it in my mouth. After about 30 seconds, I felt something different on my tongue and my throat. Desperately, I asked my friend, "Are there any peanuts in this?" "I don't know," he replied. I was really scared!

Kevin,
age 12
Allergic to peanuts
and tree nuts
Canada

I ran to my house as fast as the wind. (I knew I had an EpiPen® at school and in my house.) My friends tried to keep up with me, but I was way too fast for them. I finally arrived home. Urgently, I called my mom at work. I left a message saying, "Mom, I just ate peanuts. I'm not feeling so well. I will try to reach Grandma and Grandpa. Bye." I hung up and called my grandparents, but nobody was there. In the entrance of my house, there's a plastic bag with my EpiPen® inside. I rushed and jabbed it into the higher part of my leg. I jabbed it about three times because I wasn't sure if it had worked.

When I looked out the window, I saw my friends walking outside. I opened the door and ran outside. I tried to scream but I could barely speak. While I was running, I sort of collapsed. I saw two of my friends rushing to my house. My sisters and one of my friends went in my house and called 911. By the time my sisters and friend called 911, my other friend's mother came with her car and rushed me to the hospital.

When I arrived, they gave me a whole bunch of needles. About five minutes later, my mom arrived. She was crying. She asked me if I was okay. I said, "I'm perfectly fine, Mom." I stayed at the hospital until about 7:00 p.m.

I was really frustrated because I had missed the hockey try-outs. I still went to the arena with my dad. When I arrived, the coach asked me to go into a room. He told me that even though I had missed the try-outs, I still made the team!

So, the night started out bad, and it finished perfectly. That's my story about my peanut allergy.

About Kevin:

Siblings: Twin sisters Janelle and Josie, age 10

Career goals: NHL hockey player

Hobbies/interests: Hockey, basketball, and soccer

Editor's Note: Always read the ingredient label, even if it's a food you've eaten safely before. Additionally, never assume ingredients will be the same between different sizes of the same food.

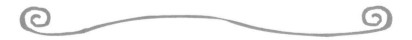

"The highest reward for a person's toil is not what they get for it, but what they become by it."

—John Rushkin

Something is Very Wrong

I have an enemy, it's not a bully or a person, much worse—a peanut!

I had been aware of my allergy since I was a year old. However it had never been never much of a problem, until I went on holiday to France when I was 8 years old. One day while we were out sightseeing, we went to McDonalds for something to eat. I ordered a chocolate sundae.

At first the girl brought me a chocolate milkshake, but my dad explained what we wanted, and she brought back a chocolate sundae—with tiny speckles of peanuts sprinkled on top–Uh oh! We took it anyway and scraped the peanuts off with a spoon (we later realized what a stupid idea this was). But what we didn't realize was that one had fallen to the bottom.

On the way back to the campsite, I was very quiet. I didn't feel 100 percent well; little did I know that a volcano inside me was getting ready to erupt. I remember it vividly, I asked my dad to bring me down to the pool, so he did.

I jumped in, even though the water was only four or five feet deep, I sank to the bottom like an anchor. I remember looking up to the surface thinking, "Oh my God, something is very wrong. How am I going to get back up there?" I did manage to get back up to the surface, and immediately asked to go back home.

Fiona,
age 15
Allergic to peanuts
Ireland

This was just the beginning; it was about a 10-minute walk back to the caravan. My body warned me just in time, because as I walked through the door, I began to have difficulty breathing and I collapsed onto the sofa. Within 10 seconds I couldn't breath at all. I turned blue and my blood pressure dropped dramatically.

When you're this close to death, all you can think of is "How will they cope?" and you begin to feel guilty that this is happening and the grief you're going to cause. Even while this was happening, I still didn't think this was the end, however the odds were not in my favor; after all I was in the middle of a campsite, hours away from a hospital, in a foreign country with no adrenaline needle. I'd been through a lot—several asthma attacks, a seizure, and a coma—but it was a little speckle of peanut that was going to kill me.

But, my parent's quick thinking saved my life. My mum put me on my nebulizer (which is used for asthma attacks), and we rushed to the nearest hospital. By the time we got there I felt fine. I was treated and kept overnight in case of a relapse.

This is something I never want to happen again, to me or to anyone. It's a terrifying experience, and definitely not worth the risk. It still upsets me today, just to think about it.

My friends are very helpful and understanding, but I think you don't fully understand the implications unless you have this condition. Awareness needs to be improved on this issue, because as long as people continue to suffer and die needlessly—it is an issue, a very serious one!

Don't let having an allergy ruin your life, improvise if you have to. If you're going out and you know people will be eating unsuitable food, eat before you go or bring some food that you love with you. And most of all, don't feel sorry for yourself; complaining helps no one, in fact it makes you feel worse, so get up and enjoy it and just get on with it—otherwise you'll go insane.

I carry epinephrine with me every where I go—it's my lifeline!

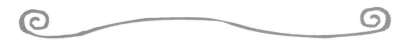

Keeping Yourself Safe

Act responsibly

Know and avoid foods and situations that pose a high risk of a reaction for you. If you are unsure if a food is safe, do not take a chance; avoid it.

Carry medicine

Keep your medications with you at all times. Be sure you understand how and when to use them.

Recognize a reaction

Know how to recognize the symptoms of an allergic reaction. Some examples include hives; swelling of the skin, lips, tongue, or throat; difficulty breathing; and vomiting.

React quickly

Have your doctor create an action plan that details what to do if you have a reaction, and follow the plan if you think you are having a reaction. If you have an EpiPen,® use it and then call for an ambulance right away. Carry your action plan with you so that you'll always know exactly what to do.

Review what happened

Talk to your doctor and parents and pinpoint ways to prevent a similar situation in the future.

If you think you are having a reaction, follow your action plan, tell someone, and get help. Going off alone, waiting to see how bad the reaction will be, or trying to drive yourself somewhere can lead to disaster.

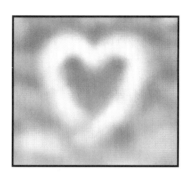

Part Three:
Growing with Food Allergies

"Each time something difficult and challenging has happened to me it has marked the beginning of a new era in my life."

-Kimberly Kirberger

Having food allergies was difficult in elementary school, but I personally think it is even harder in middle school. I just finished my first year of middle school. Boy, was that an adventure!

My family and I are very, very careful with my food allergies. We keep no peanuts in the house, and we also read the ingredients on everything I eat, even if I have eaten it before. We do that in case the company has added or changed ingredients. When I was little, I had a Medic Alert® bracelet. One cool thing about that was that a lot of people liked it and asked where I got it.

Around fifth grade, my mom decided to get me a Medic Alert® necklace instead. That way I could just wear it on the inside of my shirt, and no one had to see it. The whole point of that was so when I got older certain kids wouldn't know, because attitudes change, not always for the best.

Time moved on and I was getting ready to start middle school. My mom was very nervous. At my old school, all of the office and clinic staff and teachers knew about my allergy. Now I was going somewhere new where no one knew about it.

On registration day, I got all of the stuff I needed for a new year—my class and bus schedules, and identification. I was getting very excited. That was also the day

Cameron,
age 13
Allergic to peanuts
USA

that my mom and I met the clinic aide, Lori. She was very nice, and also very understanding. She had had several kids with peanut allergies before and knew how to handle an emergency. She also saved my mom from running around the school trying to explain my allergy to all of my teachers, by offering to tell them for us.

So, about one week later, I was all ready to start my first day of seventh grade. One thing I learned this year is that each teacher handled the information differently. My social studies teacher didn't say anything about it. I wasn't even sure he got the message.

My math teacher was very thoughtful about my allergy. One day she pulled me aside and told me that she was going to use M&Ms® for a math project. She said that it was okay, though, because she had bought plain ones, not the peanut ones. That was when I got to teach my teacher something. I explained to her that the peanut and the plain M&Ms® are made on the same equipment, and that the bag has "May contain peanuts" as part of the ingredient list. She was ecstatic about the fact that I told her. She had never known that before. That really made me feel smart. Then I suggested we use Skittles.® But she decided that it might work out for the best if the class didn't use any candy at all.

One of my biggest middle school uh-ohs was what happened in my third-period class—language arts. My language arts teacher was very nice and tried to be helpful. But, it didn't turn out that way. As she took attendance and was working on remembering names, faces, and attitudes, she got to me on the list.

She asked the usual questions about how to pronounce my name—all teachers ask those sorts of questions on the first day. Then, as she was getting ready to move on to the next kid on the list, she just had to say, "Okay, class, please remember that Cameron has a peanut allergy. Everyone be careful with peanuts around him. So, no peanuts for Cameron."

I was very embarrassed. The whole class was laughing at me. Some kids said things like, "No peanuts for Cameron!" I was laughed at for a week. I know that my teacher was only trying to help, but it was still so embarrassing. About one week later, my mom went up to the school and talked to my teacher. She explained that our family likes to keep this kind of thing private, for safety reasons. My teacher understood and apologized about mentioning it to the class.

Next, I went to science for my fourth-period class. My teacher was very understanding and kind about my allergy. If she handed out candy, she always made sure to read the ingredients, and then she even handed the bag of candy to me so I could check, in case she missed something. That worked out well.

My fifth class was computers. I didn't have to worry too much in there, because we just sat at a computer and typed, or learned how to use a program. My computer teacher didn't say anything about the allergy, and nothing involving peanuts was around. I was all set in that class.

My last class of the day was French and Spanish class. My teacher was very nice, and at the end of the semester we planned a big feast of foods from different cultures. My teacher had a very good way of letting the other students in the class know that they couldn't bring peanuts. She just said that someone in this class had a food allergy and to remember not to bring peanuts. She even asked everyone to bring the ingredient lists, just in case. We had our feast of foods from different cultures, and it was very fun.

After I came back from Christmas break, I got two new elective classes—gym and health. My mom and I went to the school on the first day back and told the new teachers about my allergy. My health teacher listened carefully, and she even asked how to use the EpiPen.® My new gym teacher didn't take the allergy too seriously, which made me very angry. I think he was just trying to be friendly and funny. The only thing is that food allergies are not funny. But eventually I got to know him, we got along fine, and I had no troubles.

The biggest fear of anyone with food allergies is the dreaded lunchroom! Our school didn't serve any kind of peanut products. That made things a little easier, since most kids buy a hot lunch. I was one of the very few that still brought my lunch. I went almost the whole year without any accidents in the lunchroom. Then, during the last week of school I had a little scare.

I was eating and talking with my friends as usual. As I was talking, using my hands as I spoke, my friends' eyes grew wide. I didn't know what had happened. Then I noticed that I had a big blob of peanut butter on my arm. My arm was already turning red. (I should also point out that my allergy is very, very severe.) I started to panic. I grabbed a napkin, wiped it off, and went to the drinking fountain to wash it off. My arm was still red. I went and sat down and finished eating my lunch. I kept an eye on my arm, the redness went down in about 10 minutes, and eventually I was okay.

As you can see, middle school is a tough neighborhood—especially for someone with food allergies. But I survived. Allergies are tough and not fun. But if you have a positive attitude, it can be a little better.

My advice to others...

Trust yourself with your allergies. No one knows them better than you.

About Cameron:

Siblings: One sister, Jacqueline

Career goals: Designer of houses or cars on a computer

Hobbies/interests: Playing on the computer and reading

"Life is about not knowing, having to change, taking the moment and making the best of it, without knowing what's going to happen next. Delicious ambiguity."

—Gilda Radner

I Have Learned to Live with Allergies

My name is Amos, and I live on a kibbutz (a settlement) in the south of Israel. Ever since I was born my parents have been very cautious about what I eat—and with good reason, too.

My dad grew up with anaphylactic allergies to eggs, nuts, fish, and mustard, and ordinary allergies to chicken, strawberries, carrots, potatoes, and many other foods. Even today, he is allergic to fish and nuts.

My parents knew that at least one of their children would have allergies. After being careful with my older brother and finding out that he does not have allergies, they were careful again, this time with me. My mother noticed that at the age of 3 months I was rubbing my limbs backward and forward against the floor. I was doing this in order to stop the itching. After I was treated with creams, which didn't work, my parents introduced me to new foods with even greater care.

On the kibbutz, all the kids under school age go to children's houses according to their age group. At the children's houses, the kids eat breakfast, lunch, and "4 o'clock snack" together. For about two years, I didn't have any problems—until I tried cheese.

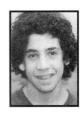

Amos,
age 16
Allergic to milk,
eggs, peanuts,
tree nuts, sesame,
and mustard
Israel

The person in charge of my children's house encouraged me to eat cottage cheese for breakfast. I remember not wanting to eat it, but I was persuaded to try it. After one bite, things turned out to be quite nasty! I went into anaphylactic shock! I was rushed by ambulance to a neighboring kibbutz where our family doctor was seeing patients. At the clinic, the doctor injected me with Ultracorten,® but unfortunately the shot did not do the trick. After the doctor phoned one of the big medical centers in the country, I was injected again, and after that I finally got life back into my system.

After the cheese incident, my parents were advised to take me to an allergy specialist. I was taken up north to meet my specialist, Dr. Dulev. He decided that having scratch tests on me could become very unpleasant and not practical because of the quantity they wanted to test. He decided to send me to a lab near the Weizmann Institute for a RAST test.

The test was going to be taken with my blood. What I didn't know was that they would fill up seven tubes with my blood! I was tested for over 150 allergens, and I tested positive for all of them, some of them with a slight reaction and some of them with a massive reaction.

My father took me to have this test done, and he said I was very brave. So on our way home, as compensation, we went to a toy shop we had visited before the test. There was a huge, blue, furry alligator, and that is what I wanted. Since then, "Agi" has lived with me, and we have a tradition that has carried on to this day. Every time I have an allergy test, I get a present, and that makes me feel good!

When we saw how many allergies I had, we had to learn how I could live with them. That meant we had to find recipes that were suitable and we had to learn how to read labels and avoid contact with milk, eggs, nuts, and peanuts. It was very hard, but we managed it. My mother had gathered recipes and the caregivers at the children's house and the children were cooperative and understanding. By the age of 5, I did not have any other reactions.

My parents knew that it would be a lot harder to keep me safe at school. On the first day of school, my father had come to my class in order to explain to my classmates that there is a special boy in their class. My classmates had to learn that they have to sit by their desks until they finished their food. School still wasn't easy.

On all the school trips, I had to have one of my parents come with me to make sure I could eat and that I wasn't in danger from everyone else's food and snacks. On the trips, I always had my medicine and my own food. It has been that way for ten years. This year was the first time that I have gone on a school trip without someone to accompany me. Of course, I still had to take my own food.

Today, I am 16 years old. I still have allergies to milk products, eggs, peanuts, and all other nuts. Wherever I go, I carry my medicine. Every night I take medicine to control my asthma. That's a great improvement! I used to take as many as four medications four times a day. I have never allowed my allergies to stop me from being like a normal kid. At school I participate in gym class and I get good results. I have won medals in track and tennis and I love to play baseball and ultimate Frisbee.® One day a week I work in our experimental orchards, where we grow exotic fruits.

My allergies have always made me feel special, and at times I have even bragged about them. I have learned to live with my allergies, but there is still room for improvement, especially with my surroundings. In conclusion, I do not have trouble with my allergies, only with the people who turn my allergies into a problem.

About Amos...

Siblings: One brother, Nisan, age 21, one sister, Gavriella, age 12

Career goals: Making the world a better place for himself

Hobbies/interests: Playing tennis and baseball, and running

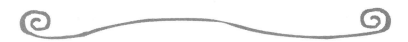

I have had allergies all of my life. I found out when I was 11 months old, when I ate a peanut butter cookie. Ever since then, my parents and I have been very careful. Wherever we go, we always bring an EpiPen® and read the ingredients in whatever I eat.

Here are some tips that I've learned along the way.

- I have found that the easiest way to read ingredient labels is to look at the last ingredient first, before reading the rest of the ingredients. I do this because that is usually where you can find a "May contain peanuts" message. If it is not there, then I continue to read the rest of the ingredients.

- I make sure I look to see that no one near me is eating peanut butter when I am eating lunch.

- When we are flying in an airplane, we always call ahead and make sure that they are not serving any peanuts.

- If someone else in school offers me food, I ask if there is a list of ingredients. If not, I do not eat it. If they keep telling me it's okay, I tell them I am not hungry and they leave me alone.

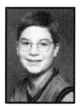

- Almond oil is in some soaps and shampoos.

Paul,
age 12
Allergic to peanuts
USA

Sometimes I wish I could walk into a restaurant and without reading the ingredients, eat whatever I want. Or go into a chocolate shop and try all of the samples.

Sometimes I wish that I could just switch bodies with someone for a day. I would go to all of the ice cream shops, chocolate shops, and restaurants in my town. I would also not have to read any of the ingredients of any food that I eat.

I hope that someday my wish will come true.

My advice to others...

Don't stop reading ingredients, and always carry your EpiPen® with you.

About Paul...

Siblings: One sister, Clare, age 11

Career goals: Astronaut or marine biologist

Hobbies/Interests: Basketball, soccer, swimming, music, saxophone

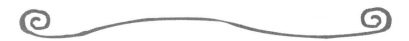

$\mathcal{B}$efore I overcame my fear of peanuts, I felt that I was very different. My perception was that my whole life centered on my allergy. When I was around 7 or 8 years old, I would introduce myself to someone new by saying, "Hi, I'm Len. I have a peanut allergy." I identified myself by my allergy.

Through the years, I have changed quite a lot about the way I deal with peanuts. In first and second grade, I ate lunch at a mini-table on a stage in the cafeteria. It certainly drew attention to my food allergy. In third grade, I mingled at a table with children selected to sit with me due to the fact that they didn't bring peanut butter. In fourth grade at a new school, I went back to sitting at a separate, small table due to my fears that the table on which I ate could be contaminated with peanuts.

When I came back to school the next year, I felt I didn't need my little table and was comfortable sitting at the end seat with a group of my friends. In sixth grade, I found a comfortable position to take on the issue of lunch in school. I mingled with friends at a regular table.

Another event that helped me a lot was a three-week sleep-away summer camp I attended when I was 11. By making food choices every day in the absence of my parents' help, I gained confidence in my own decisions concerning food. The next year a different camp allowed me

Len,
age 13
Allergic to peanuts, legumes, soy, and tree nuts
USA

to feel really safe on my own, but for different reasons. The kitchen staff served my food whether it was safe or not. On one occasion, they served food that was unsafe, then refused to recognize that I couldn't eat it. They just didn't "get it."

From being a kid scared silly of peanuts, I am now an independent and food-conscious teenager. I always carry EpiPen®s and Benadryl.® And I like who I am.

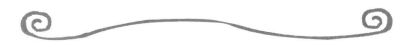

Taking Control

$\mathcal{G}$ rowing up with food allergies is a difficult thing for any person to deal with. You can feel left out or isolated from your peers in school. You cannot share in the pizza parties or birthday parties that are so frequent in grammar and middle school. You don't feel comfortable going over to friends' houses or restaurants because you cannot fully control your surroundings. You are always struggling for responsibility while your parents try to keep an eye on you. Wherever you go, day or night, you always have to keep your guard up and be aware of what is going on, a difficult thing for any person to do.

Elementary and middle school can seem to be the hardest thing to handle for a young kid. Every time you go to lunch, you have to ask the teacher if the food is okay. Other kids label you as Billy-the-kid-who-can't-have-pizza or Sally-the-girl-who-can't-eat-a-peanut-butter-and-jelly-sandwich. Kids will do cruel things like leave a peanut in your lunch box or spit milk at you just to see what will happen.

You can feel left out or segregated from the other kids when you just want to fit in. As hard as it feels, you must realize that you do fit in, but you just have to be a little aware of the food you eat. Everyone has their problems in life, but food allergies are something that can be controlled.

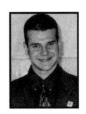

Joe,
age 22
Allergic to peanuts
and tree nuts
USA

High school can be the most exciting, stressful, and frustrating time in your life. You are trying to deal with passing your classes, making new friends, learning how to drive, and going to parties. But teens who have food allergies have to be more careful than other kids in normal everyday situations. One of the hardest things to accomplish is trying to get your parents to relax. You are becoming an adult and you want more responsibility, but they are reluctant because of your food allergies.

What you need to do is actually show them that you are responsible and can make decisions as an adult. You need to work with your doctor to develop an emergency plan and explain to your parents what you would do in an emergency situation, for instance, if you were out with your friends. Your friends need to be trained in your emergency plan and in how to use an EpiPen.® This can be hard to do, but, when you find your true group of friends, they will accept you for who you are and not judge you based solely on your food allergies.

For me, growing up with food allergies was a hard thing to deal with. Kids always separated me, labeled me, and made fun of me because of my food allergies. They just did not realize how serious a problem it was—that one little bite could kill me. Grammar and middle school were especially hard, but, as time went on, it got easier.

In high school, people are a little bit older, more mature, and open-minded. Friends at lunch used to make sure that the food was okay and kept an eye on me. It was when I found my true group of friends that I found handling my food allergies easier. I began to see that people accepted me for who I was and, when aware of my food allergies, still accepted me. You will find that people will accept you for the person you are, allergies included.

When you get to adulthood, you begin to realize what role food allergies play in your life. You know that you have to control them and not let them control you.

When I was growing up, there were no support groups or organizations dedicated to helping people with food allergies. I thought that I was the only kid in the world with food allergies. Eventually, I realized that I was not alone and that I could be like any other person: I could run, play, and so on, but I just couldn't eat everything that others did. You will learn that people are curious about you and want to know more about you and your food allergies.

As each day goes by, you have the potential to educate someone about food allergies—that is a great thing.

My advice to others...

Everyone has their own problems in life—those with food allergies just have to watch the foods that they eat. Be the person that you want to be, but be prepared and stay safe.

About Joe...

Siblings: None

Career goals: Pharmacist

Hobbies/Interests: Running, mountain biking, and water-skiing. Joe has moderated teen sessions at FAAN's Food Allergy Conferences. He answers questions from teens with food allergies on the "He Says…She Says…" page of the FANTEEN website, www.fanteen.org.

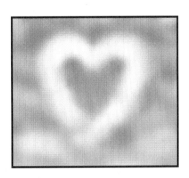

Part Four: Acceptance

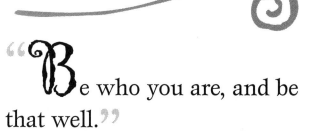

"Be who you are, and be that well."

−St. Francis de Sales

I have had food allergies for as long as I can remember. I really don't think anything bad about my food allergies—they are just a part of me that's unique. I have learned to accept my food allergies as life; that helps me resist the foods that cause me to have an anaphylactic reaction. I've only had one or two reactions that I can remember, and at least one was from cross contact.

That's just one of the things that's hard about food allergies. Many people don't realize the severity of food allergies, or they just don't care enough to take the extra effort to check the ingredients. It is hard to go to new places to eat because a lot of restaurants just don't understand how to manage food allergies. Even going places where I have eaten before is hard because I have to check the ingredients each time, in case the manufacturer changes the ingredients.

That is another hard thing for me, since I have multiple food allergies. Many manufacturers don't point out that the product could have cross contact with another item. I just can't feel totally safe eating manufactured foods.

Krista,
age 13
Allergic to eggs,
peanuts, tree nuts,
fish, and shellfish
USA

Food allergies haven't prevented me from doing the things I want to do. I have gone to many different camps and stayed away from home anywhere from two to seven days. I usually pack my own food for those times when I can't eat what others are eating. At home, I have found some foods to replace the foods I can't eat, such as soy butter instead of peanut butter. Another substitution we use is a special mixture of water, oil, and baking powder to replace the egg in some baked goods we make at home. We have been collecting lots of dessert recipes to use.

There are many setbacks for me when it comes to eating, but I'm glad that my friends are always there for me. At home, I have two younger brothers. The youngest, Gregory, doesn't have any food allergies, but the other, Jason, is allergic to eggs, peanuts, and tree nuts. They both help me avoid my allergens, and I help Jason with his allergies.

At school, my teachers know about my allergies, along with the lunch lady, the school nurse, and my classmates. My friends help me most by treating me normally, because they know I really don't like sympathy. They also help me by checking some ingredients for me, and not offering foods to me that don't have ingredient labels.

I know it isn't easy to live with food allergies (trust me!), but thanks to my family, teachers, friends, and all the other understanding and caring people out there, I can live a little easier knowing I'm cared for.

About Krista...

Siblings: Two brothers, Jason and Gregory

Career Goals: Marine biologist

Hobbies/Interests: Playing soccer, basketball, and volleyball, and being a Cadette Girl Scout

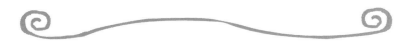

"Never underestimate the power of dreams and the influence of the human spirit. We are all the same in this notion: The potential for greatness lives within each of us."

—Wilma Rudolph

I Can't Change It

Although I have had a wheat allergy since I was about 10 years old, I am still learning more every day how to live with it. I have never been able to grab a piece of pizza while out with friends. I can't eat a burger on school trips or camps like everyone else.

Being allergic to wheat, especially as a teen, is not at all fun or easy. It's hard to avoid wheat, especially with foods today. It is very tempting at times, but I know my limits.

I have learned how to live without wheat in my life. I have learned that I can make some foods myself. I just have to make food from scratch and substitute wheat-free ingredients for wheat ingredients. I also eat things that I can to meet my needs. I am hooked on Mexican food. I think of rice cakes as cookies.

I think that being allergic to wheat has made me more of an independent person as well as a stronger person. I don't always have to follow the crowd and do what everyone else does all the time.

Sometimes, though, I don't like being so different; I just want to be like everyone else and have a fun life. Being allergic to wheat can be depressing at times. It's affected my life in the ways I think of myself and others. I have tried to blame my allergy on other people. I have blamed the fact that I can't eat bread on the

Kristie,
age 17
Allergic to wheat
USA

people who eat it right in front of me. This was more of jealousy than anything else, though.

All of the depression, temptation, and jealousy changed after I had a severe allergic reaction. My last reaction was very severe. I ate chicken one day before work. I did not realize or even think about the fact that the chicken was breaded. After about an hour of working, I started itching and turning red. I went home and passed out in my mother's arms. The next day, I made an appointment with an allergist. I then realized that I was allergic to wheat and that I could not ever change that.

I became a member of the Food Allergy & Anaphylaxis Network and found recipe ideas. I no longer have the desire to eat wheat products. I have found that I can have fun in life and have a good time even without pizza and burgers. I once heard a saying: "It's not the things you go through in life that matter; it's how you handle them."

My mom found out I was allergic to peanuts when I was about 15 months old. My mom's friend came over and said to give me a cracker with some peanut butter on it. My mom had never considered giving me peanut butter at such a young age, but since her friend had given her son some and he loved it, she decided to give me some. I don't remember anything because I was so young, but I was told I loved it. My mom and I were both eating it together, with me sitting on her lap.

A short time later my grandfather, who was changing my diaper, noticed I had red lines around my mouth. He called my parents in, and within minutes my face had swollen up so much that I looked like a prizefighter who had lost the fight. Then I was having problems breathing.

My dad immediately put me in the car, and we were on our way to the hospital. The doctors told my parents I had an allergic reaction, and since I was eating peanut butter when it happened, it was the peanuts. When my mom held me after the doctors worked on me, I started to react all over again.

Apparently when I was sitting on her lap eating the peanut butter, I had gotten some in her hair. When she held me, my face touched her hair where some peanut butter was. The doctors told my mom to wash

Tim,
age 14
Allergic to peanuts
USA

her hair right there in the hospital before she could hold me again.

I was told to avoid peanuts, peanut butter, and anything cooked in peanut oil. When I was three, I was re-tested by an allergist. The test showed that I was majorly allergic to peanuts, and I would never outgrow it. So no peanut butter and jelly sandwiches for me.

It's been very hard being allergic to peanuts. They seem to be everywhere—on planes, at parties, in school, and in candy. If there are no peanuts in something, it is made with the same utensils or near something that has peanuts, so I can't eat it. No more chocolate doughnuts or Nestlé Crunch® bars. I used to love them, but now the ingredients say, "May contain nuts."

The allergist said I can eat other nuts, but I am afraid to. I also don't like people to eat peanuts near me. I'm probably wrong in this, but I'm just scared. My good friends won't eat anything with peanuts in front of me. But I do have friends that do. And I feel bad when their parents get upset with me, and don't understand the way I feel, and tell me I am paranoid. I'm not eating it, they say, so don't worry about it. I really like it when my friends' parents understand and won't have peanuts around.

People need to be more educated about peanut allergy—such as restaurants. I hate it when the waiter has no idea what oil they cook their food in.

As far as school is concerned, kids can be really mean. I don't like to tell anyone except my close friends because they will throw peanuts at me or try to smash me with their peanut butter sandwiches. Teachers are also not well educated about allergies. Sometimes when we do something good, the teacher will reward us with a candy bar. Most of the time, it's a Butterfinger® or Snickers® bar.

I think the worst part of this is that I feel so alone. I don't know anyone else who is allergic to peanuts like I am. Everyone I know can eat anything they want and not have to worry. Me, I have to read the ingredients on everything, plus carry an EpiPen.®

Eating is a way of life, and this should not happen to anyone. Hopefully someday they will find a cure for this so I can be like the rest of the kids.

My advice to others...

Be careful what you eat, read the ingredients, and carry your EpiPen.® There could be worse things in life than having a food allergy.

About Tim...

Siblings: Two step-brothers and one step-sister

Career goals: Doctor or actor

Hobbies/Interests: Riding his dirt bike and moped

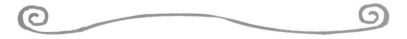

"Opportunities are usually disguised as hard work, so most people don't recognize them."

—Ann Landers

When I was 13, my parents and I at last discovered that an undiagnosed milk allergy had been causing my mysterious medical symptoms. Someone once had the nerve to say to me, "I might have to shoot myself if I couldn't eat ice cream or pizza!" I, however, gladly eliminated from my diet the elements that had caused me so much embarrassment.

It was hard, but religiously scrutinizing food labels seemed a minute exchange for the freedom it gave me to breathe. Unfortunately, 13 years of awkwardness had already passed in time. Incomplete school days and curious glances still lingered in my consciousness, my dreams, my nightmares, and my hopes.

I am at Max's Opera Café now, with some friends I've made at college this quarter. We laugh and talk and something I say stirs up a little laughter. The sign of acceptance means more than they will ever know.

"Are you ready to order?"

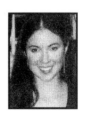

Not again. What order were my questions in again? I'm not really in the mood for another biology lesson. Can't I ever just... "I'll have the ham sandwich. Can I have that on sourdough bread instead of French? Can you make sure that it's not cooked in butter? Okay,

Serena,
age 18
Allergic to milk
USA

that's fine then. And there's no cheese in this right? Well, is the coleslaw dairy-free? What about the potato salad?...No, that's fine. And the Italian soda, there's no cream in that, right? Okay, then that's it."

The normal question-and-answer session follows. Yes, cheese is a dairy product. No, I can't have pizza. Yes, that means ice cream, too. No, lactose is the milk sugar. I'm allergic to the milk protein...right, that means I can't take that pill-thingy. Yes, I've tried it. No, I can't drink Lactaid.® No, I will not have some anyway. It's really not a huge deal!

They will say things to me like "Come on, a little piece of cheese won't hurt," and on road trips, "So, where are all the places you can't eat again?" But they don't realize that we are speaking two separate languages.

Over time, I have come to realize that a unique food allergy is not only interesting but gives newly acquainted groups a topic to discuss. It's an icebreaker. I'm not as defensive as I used to be about the subject. It used to conjure up bad memories of my mother and me in the bathroom with my head over the toilet, trying to clear my lungs of the allergic reaction that had remained undiagnosed. Or sometimes I thought of the cute boy named Jacob in my first-grade class who asked me to "stop snoring" during story time when I was only breathing. My allergic episodes wounded a portion of my self-esteem for several years, but gradually I have learned to deal with these feelings and then put them behind me.

Growing up as a "sickly child" has shaped me, but it does not define me. I should be thankful that knowledge of my allergy has enabled me to lead a healthy life. I shouldn't get so antsy about explaining my allergy to others. I will instead see it as an opportunity to remind myself daily of how grateful I am.

Every morning when I awake, I thank God for creating me. And then, do I ask God why He let "that" happen to me when I was younger? Sure I do. Have I asked God why He did not obliterate my symptoms when they first appeared? Sure I have. But I also know that because of them I am stronger.

Instances that might not have mattered make much larger impressions. Would I want to be a doctor if I had not experienced the pain of sickness? Could I feel as much? Could I appreciate as much? Could I love as much? God did not abandon me to sickness but instead carried me through it and changed my future.

But when the waiter leaves and the questions begin, I know my friends will scarcely understand the medical terminology, let alone the spiritual implications, of my milk allergy. And so the night moves forward, as I wonder inside whether food creates deep emotions in others, as it does in me. I know I am not the only one with a story. We each carry our food preferences to the table of food, and our experiences to the table of life. And, despite our differences, I tend to think that they are all related.

My advice to others...

Try not to get down on yourself about "all the things wrong with you," and focus on the life you have and the talents that have been given to you.

About Serena...

Siblings: One sister, Carley, age 20

Career goals: To pursue a doctorate in neuropsychology, and teach

Hobbies/interests: Performing music, watching independent and foreign movies, making jewelry, acting, hiking, going to and helping out at church, hanging out with friends, and finding sweets that are milk-free

"Hey, you're the girl with the problems!"

It's 5 o'clock, and I'm riding home from dance practice with my friend and her new boyfriend. As soon as he blurts out this random thought, his face turns red and I can see his regret for vocalizing the ridiculous statement. "Yes, I am the girl with the problems. Nice to meet you," I say, smiling despite myself. When this boy so subtly reminds me of my claim to fame at our high school, I do not feel embarrassed or insulted. I am, by now, used to my circumstance.

Ever since I was an infant, I have had terrible food allergies. While other children were struggling to say "Ma-ma" and "Pa-pa," at a moment's notice I could name at least 10 words as large as sodium caseinate. It seemed as if with every growth spurt, more foods were added to my list of allergies. By the time I reached middle school, I was tall, spindly, and able to name just about every hospital in New England.

Knowing that accidental ingestion of certain foods could kill me, I was forced to grow up and take complete responsibility for myself. At 11 years old, I was mature enough to make life-or-death decisions. Is this restaurant a safe environment, or is there a chance of cross contact with my dinner?

Tina,
age 17
Allergic to peanuts, tree nuts, and sesame and poppy seeds (outgrew milk allergy)
USA

Should I trust Auntie when she tells me that there is no milk or peanuts in the apple pie? Does my situation necessitate the use of an EpiPen®? Even as a middle schooler, I was prepared to give myself a shot if needed.

As time went on, my allergies seemed only to get worse. Eventually, even smelling certain foods made me ill. For six years, half of my public education, I was not able to eat in any school cafeteria. Being isolated each afternoon while others ate lunch and being ostracized by classmates because they weren't allowed to bring food into the classrooms were difficult burdens.

It did not take long for me to realize, however, that my food allergies did not have to define me. I worked hard in school and excelled in extracurricular activities to counter this void in my life. Having food allergies helped me realize one of my strongest personality traits: the strength to overcome adversity. Even though nature seemed to be against me, I conquered my allergies by living the most normal life that I could. I attended school regularly, maintained good grades, played sports, and immersed myself in the arts.

Thankfully, after years of careful management, my food allergies gradually decreased in severity. Looking back, I can only hope that sharing my experiences with food allergies will inspire other teenagers, not only to overcome adversity in their lives but also to thrive in its path.

About Tina...

Siblings: One brother, Nick, age 8

Career goals: Broadcast journalism

Hobbies/interests: Dancing, singing, and acting

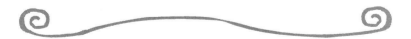

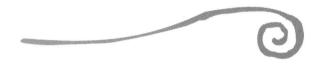

"A pessimist is one who makes difficulties of his opportunities; an optimist is one who makes opportunities of his difficulties."

–Reginald B. Mansell

A Way of Life

All my life, my body has dictated to me where I can go and what I can do, especially when it comes to eating. And since I love food, this can sometimes be a problem.

Not being able to eat certain foods never really bothered me until I found out what it was that I was missing. I didn't care that I couldn't eat real ice cream; I ate fruit sorbet instead. That's what I thought ice cream was, until I attended my first birthday party.

When it was time for cake and ice cream, I was confused because what they were serving wasn't ice cream—it was all creamy and brown, not icy and pink like what I was used to. So I asked what it was that they were serving. Everyone laughed at me and said, "That's ice cream, silly! Haven't you ever seen ice cream before?" When I shook my head, they laughed again. That's when I knew that I was different.

After that party, it really bothered me that I couldn't eat the same things as everyone else. I couldn't buy school lunches, couldn't eat dinner at my friends' houses, and couldn't have a lot of snacks there either. The ice cream man came and left me empty-handed when all my friends were devouring their humongous cones of dripping, sweet, frozen confections. And what bothered me most of all was

Jessica,
age 17
Allergic to milk, soy,
peanuts, and shellfish
USA

that I couldn't eat the same dinner as my family. When they have steaks, I have chicken. If everyone is munching on eggs, I have a bagel.

For the longest time, that really annoyed me, until I matured a little, took a step back, and looked at the big picture. Okay, I realized, so maybe I can't eat a couple of foods. Big deal. There are people out there who are much worse off than I am. I can breathe on my own, run, jump, skip, and turn cartwheels. Most of all, I'm alive.

I vowed not to let food allergies run my life. I refuse to even acknowledge the fact that having food allergies is considered a "handicap," because it's not. It's just something I have to deal with; it's a way of life. No matter where we go, there's always something I can eat, and I am thankful for that.

So perhaps what having food allergies has given me is simply the ability to be grateful for what I do have and what I can do. I have a wide circle of friends, I am a cheerleader and an honor student, and I have a very supportive family.

Life is life, and you can't change that. God only gives people what they can handle, and I know for sure that I've got this one covered.

About Jessica...

Siblings: Two brothers, Michael, age 14, and Matthew, age 7

Career goals: To own and operate a business in psychology or communication

Hobbies/interests: Cheerleading, reading, writing, shopping, swimming, and laying on the beach

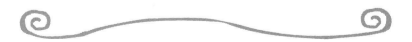

"You must be the change you wish to see in the world."

−Mahatma Gandhi

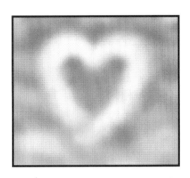

Part Five: How One Person Can Make a Difference

"Out of respect for things that I was never destined to do, I have learned that my strengths are a result of my weaknesses, my success is due to my failures, and my style is directly related to my limitations."

—Billy Joel

People Do Care

On a snowy day in March, 16 years ago, I was born. I weighed only 5 pounds, 11 ounces. Since I was so small, my father decided to give me the nickname "peanut." Little did he know that when I was 2, they would discover my allergy to peanuts! I guess I really didn't like that name!

One day at school, during math class, my new friend Bryan* was hungry. So he pulled out a bag of peanuts. Quickly, I simply asked him not to eat them. Confused, he said, "Why? They are healthy. They are good for me."

My friend Aidan* came to my side and said, "Well, they aren't healthy for Larissa. She's allergic to them." Hearing this, Bryan quickly put them away and excused himself. When he returned, we asked him where he had run off to. He told us that he had gone to the bathroom to wash his hands.

Aidan asked him, "Why did you do that? You didn't even eat any." Bryan said, "But there could have been peanutty stuff on the outside of the bag. I didn't want to kill Larissa, so I figured I would wash my hands."

It was then I realized that people are informed about allergies and that they do care. It is really easy to simply ask a person not to eat something while you are around. It is not easy to tell them once you are having trouble breathing and getting hives.

Larissa,
age 16
Allergic to peanuts
Canada

Names have been changed.

My advice to others...

Never be afraid to ask; it's your life in jeopardy, not theirs. If the person refuses to understand your reasons, just leave the room.

About Larissa...

Siblings: One brother Daniel, age 15

Career goals: High school teacher

Hobbies/Interests: Swimming, badminton, and reading

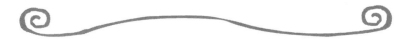

I have had many experiences with my food allergies, both good and bad, but I'm sure you would rather hear about some of the good ones.

Once when I was staying at a hotel, I wasn't able to eat many of the breakfasts. So, every day, the cook would make me something special or I would go into the kitchen and help make my own breakfast. I think it's great that some people are so thoughtful and adaptable.

One night my family was having dinner at a nice restaurant. Before we left, I went into the washroom with my mom, and saw a lady who was having a lot of trouble breathing. It turned out that she was having an anaphylactic reaction to some food she had just eaten. She didn't know that she had anaphylaxis so she didn't have an EpiPen.®

In the end she used mine and immediately began to recover. Then we called for an ambulance, and she went to the hospital. I've often thought about how amazing it was that we happened to walk into that washroom just as she needed help.

Aisling,
age 11
Allergic to peanuts,
tree nuts, chickpeas,
and soy
Canada

My advice to others...

Don't let your allergies hold you back. Always check labels and be careful. If you're having trouble, don't go off on your own; get help.

About Aisling...

Siblings: One brother Gareth, age 8, and one sister Aife, age 4

Career goals: Theatre actress and art and history teacher

Hobbies/Interests: Acting, singing, painting, drawing, snowboarding, swimming, helping out at a center for handicapped children, and shopping

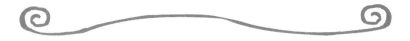

The Day I Saved the Director

One day in June, I went to school. As usual, we had math, then science, after that French, and finally lunch. So I went to these classes and then went to daycare for lunch. That day for lunch we were having egg rolls, and Judith (the director) was serving the food.

When I finished my lunch, I realized that Judith had hives and was having trouble breathing. Since I have experienced the same thing before, I asked her three questions: "What are you allergic to? Do you have an EpiPen®? Do you know how to use an EpiPen®?"

She answered, "I am allergic to peanuts and shellfish. Yes, I do have an EpiPen,® but, no, I do not know how to use it."

"No? You don't know how to use an EpiPen®!? Well, I'll have to teach you!" I yelled. "First, you must take off the gray cap, then jab the EpiPen® into your thigh." So she did that, and then I told her, "All you have to do is wait 10 seconds."

Judith asked, "That's it?"

"No, go directly to the hospital!" I hastily replied.

So two people took Judith to the hospital, and I went to class.

The next day when I went to daycare, Judith was serving the food again.

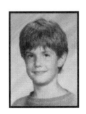

David,
age 11
Allergic to
peanuts and soy
Canada

About David...

Siblings: Twin sisters Emma and Laura, age 9

Career goals: Aerospace engineer or scientist

Hobbies/Interests: Downhill and cross country skiing, fishing, soccer, and chess

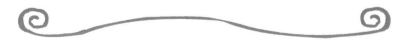

Hi, my name is Alex and I am now 11 years old. I am allergic to peas, beans, nuts, sesame seeds, and fish. I have known about these allergies for nine years, and I have also learned that you shouldn't always judge a book by its cover. Here is why.

During Easter, I was on a cruise ship sailing toward the Norwegian fjords (which are narrow valleys of sea between cliffs). I woke up one morning not knowing that it was going to be a day that I would always remember. I walked to the breakfast hall and decided to try what looked like a bowl of ordinary cereal, just like the ones I have at home. It was served in a glass bowl.

I was happily munching away when my lips started to feel rather dodgy. Next, my tummy felt like it was being pressed against the table. "Mum, I feel sick!" I groaned. Then I "legged it" to the toilet. After I was sick, my mum took me to the sick bay on the ship, where they worked their magic and I got better.

Afterward, the nurse got the box of cereal and tried to check the ingredients. However, to her and most of the crew, it was all gobble-de-gook! Luckily we finally found someone who told us it was written in Arabic and that they could read it. It turned out that the cereal I had

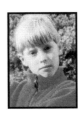

Alex,
age 11
Allergic to peas,
beans, tree nuts,
sesame seeds, and fish
United Kingdom

eaten contained nuts and wasn't the cereal I was used to having at home.

We reported the incident, and because of me the cruise line now has nut warnings on every food counter and does not take the cereals out of the boxes.

So, on the day I remember, it turned out that one person, age 10, changed all the food labeling systems on this cruise line!

About Alex...

Siblings: None

Career goals: To make money to buy lots of computer games

Hobbies/Interests: Playing Playstation® and Gameboy®

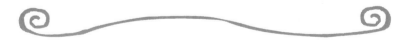

Opportunities to Educate

*H*ave you ever wished that you could share more about food allergies with your classmates without feeling awkward? A lot of times, school projects give us a unique opportunity to tell others about our allergies without stepping out of our comfort zones.

I've used opportunities in college to teach my peers about food allergies. Even though I'm very shy in person, I've still found ways to share information about my problem. Maybe my experiences will inspire you to do something similar in school.

For oral interpretation (a class that involves reading the written word with interpretive emotion), I read a newspaper article about a woman whose daughter is severely allergic to peanuts. After I was finished reading, one of the students who was in attendance told our class a bit about a professor at our college who suffers from a severe peanut allergy— something I had not known before! Sharing about your food allergies may lead to your finding out that other people have them, too.

For a fiction-writing class in which we did peer reviews, I wrote about a girl who was made fun of in school because of her food allergies. While in a store with her friend, she got so embarrassed at being made fun of that she ate foods she

Melissa,
age 22
Allergic to milk,
eggs, peanuts, soy,
and wheat
USA

was allergic to in front of the students and got severely sick. This story was therapeutic for me, because so many times I've felt the same way (wanting to cheat on my diet and be "normal"). It also prompted students to ask me more about my problem and what it is like to live with food allergies. Sharing about your food allergies may lead to an informative discussion.

A lot of us complain about how little our peers know about food allergies. But we belong to this generation, and it's our responsibility to teach others about them. I used to hide my food allergies from other students, but I learned that it's much better to be open about our problems so that we can educate others.

About Melissa...

Siblings: One brother, Daniel, age 24

Career goals: Writer or editor

Hobbies/interests: Writing, reading, animals, karaoke, and drawing

Thanks, Mom!

I am a 13-year-old who is anaphylactic to nuts and peanuts; I have had this allergy since the age of 2. I have found that since I've been in school it has been a little scary, and it will get even scarier when I get into high school. Although I have only had three anaphylactic reactions, there have been some close calls. I have found that one way to avoid coming into contact with the things I'm allergic to at school is not to share snacks, and in science class I wear gloves to be on the safe side.

One person who has stuck by me since I got my allergy is my mom; she is always there. We are like the closest friends ever. My mom always understands when I need help, and she's there by my hospital bed when I need her. I can always count on her. One thing that everyone should know is that, even though you may have 100 heroes, moms like mine are heroes, too.

In conclusion, I would like to say that if my mom wasn't there for me, then and now, for my allergy, I don't know where I'd be. Thanks, Mom!

About Marie-Claire...

Siblings: Two sisters, Courtney, age 13 and Emilie-Ann, age 11

Career goals: Teacher or translator

Hobbies/Interests: Playing the piano, singing, reading, and swimming

Marie-Claire,
age 13
Allergic to peanuts
and tree nuts
Canada

"The only real mistake is the one from which we learn nothing."

—John Powell

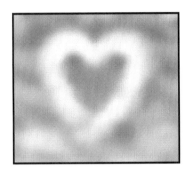

How Savvy Are You About Food Allergy Management?

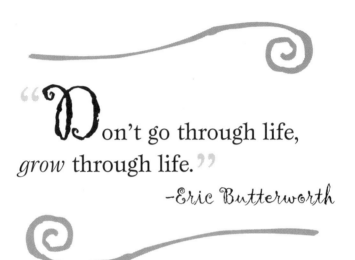

"Don't go through life, *grow* through life."

—Eric Butterworth

How Savvy Are You About Food Allergy Management?

1. Your friend, who has known about your peanut allergy since elementary school, has brought a batch of homemade brownies to school and wants you to try one. Upon close inspection, you don't see any peanuts. You decide to…

   A. *touch a brownie to your tongue to see if it will tingle as a method to determine whether the brownies are safe for you to eat.*

   B. *tell your friend you know he or she means well and understands your allergy, but you don't want to risk having a reaction.*

   C. *call your mom or dad and ask if it's okay to eat.*

2. You are in a rush to meet your friends at the mall. You grab a quick snack, and glance at the ingredient label as you eat the food. By the time you get to the mall, you are feeling nauseous. You aren't sure that it has anything to do with the snack you ate. You handle this by…

   A. *waiting a little bit to see if your symptoms will get worse.*

   B. *telling your friends you'll catch up with them a little later and driving yourself home.*

   C. *deciding that there is a good chance that this is a reaction and following your doctor's instructions for treatment.*

3. You are surveying the food set out in serving dishes at a party, and you notice there aren't any ingredient labels available. Everyone around you is eating and that makes you want to do the same. You…

   A. pick the food that "looks" the safest.

   B. grab something to drink so you aren't just standing around.

   C. try to find the bag the food came in so you could read the label.

4. You are at the university dining hall and it's teeming with students. You notice a dessert being served that you have safely eaten before. Since it appears to be the same dessert, you…

   A. order it, but eat it slowly.

   B.. ask the server what's in it.

   C. skip dessert.

5. You're at a restaurant with a group of friends, including someone you'd like to go out with. You order your burger without cheese. A few minutes later, your meal arrives, and there is cheese on your burger. You…

   A. ask the server to fix you a new burger.

   B. eat everything except the burger because you don't want to make a big deal.

   C. peel the cheese away and don't eat the part of the bun that had cheese on it.

6. You and two friends are planning on catching a movie this afternoon. You are running late, and you can't remember where you've put your EpiPen.® Your friends are impatiently waiting for you, so you decide to…

   A. look for it later; after all, you don't plan on eating anything.

   B. tell your friends they'll have to wait while you find it, or tell them to go ahead without you and make arrangements to meet them there.

   C. go without it and figure you can buy medicine at the drugstore if you need it.

7. You are going to a movie with a friend. Before the movie starts, the two of you look around the concession stand. Among the bins of candy, you notice a double bin—one side is filled with chocolate-covered peanuts and the other side is filled with chocolate covered raisins. You are allergic to peanuts, but you love raisins. You decide to…

   A. buy the chocolate-covered raisins.

   B. pass on the bulk candy; there is too high a risk of cross contact with the chocolate-covered peanuts.

   C. figure it's okay to eat the raisins; if you have a reaction, your friend will probably know what to do.

8. A trip to the beach is in the works. You plan to…

A. keep your meds in an insulated bag to protect them from the heat, sun, and sand.

B. leave your meds in the car, figuring you probably won't need them at the shore.

C. leave your meds at home because you aren't planning on eating anything.

9. You are planning a camping trip with your scouting troop. You…

A. don't plan to bring your meds with you; instead, you'll carry a cell phone, just in case.

B. practice what to do in the event of an emergency by showing your troop leaders and friends what they can do to help you and where they can find your medicine.

C. pack all your own food and tell yourself that because you aren't planning on eating anything else, there is no need to worry.

10. At a friend's house last week, you ate something without reading the ingredient label and had a reaction. You treated the reaction and decided not to tell your parents about it. Later, when your friend called your house to ask how you were, your parents found out, and now they are upset. You handle the situation by…

A. refusing to talk about it; after all, you took care of the problem, and there is no cause for alarm.

B. explaining to your parents why you weren't up-front with them about your reaction.

C. yelling and screaming; the louder you are, the more your parents will take you seriously.

How Did You Do?

1. The answer is B: If this is a true friend, there won't be any hard feelings. He or she will understand that you don't want to risk having a reaction.

Did you answer A? "Taste testing" is not an accurate way to determine whether a food contains an ingredient to which you are allergic; in fact, severe reactions have occurred because of this practice.

Did you answer C? Your mom and dad didn't bake the brownies, and since there isn't an ingredient label available, they won't be able to tell you if the brownies are safe for you to eat.

2. The answer is C: By quickly glancing at an ingredient label, it's possible that you missed something. Always read the label before you eat the food; reading the label as you are eating the product could be dangerous.

Did you answer A? By waiting to see if you will have other symptoms, you are losing precious time to treat a reaction before it gets out of hand.

Did you answer B? Because a reaction can quickly get out of control, you shouldn't be driving.

3. The answer is B: If there isn't an ingredient label for a food, don't take a chance. Eat before you go to the party, and stick with something to drink to be on the safe side.

Did you answer A? You cannot tell just by looking at something whether it contains a food you should avoid. Additionally, in a party setting, cross contact between foods on the table is always a danger.

Did you answer C? The risk of matching up the wrong food to the wrong bag is too high.

4. The answer is C: Desserts are high risk; the potential for them to contain an ingredient to which you are allergic is high.

Did you answer A? Eating slowly doesn't prevent a reaction, nor will it give you more time to determine whether symptoms will appear. Don't take the chance!

Did you answer B? Desserts are often prepared off-site for food service establishments (i.e., dining halls and restaurants), and although the server may have access to the ingredient label, keep in mind that he or she will likely not know about possible cross contact with the food you are avoiding during its preparation.

5. The answer is A: Ask the server to fix you a new burger. Keep the first burger at the table with you until the new one arrives. This will ensure that the cheese isn't simply removed from the original one, and that the same burger won't be presented to you as a new one.

Did you answer B? Although this might be an option, keeping quiet won't teach the restaurant staff anything. Use this opportunity to practice being assertive. Consider creating a "chef card" for the server to pass on to the chef so that he or she will have a written reminder of the ingredients you need to avoid. A sample chef card is pictured here.

Sample Chef Card

To the Chef:

WARNING! I am allergic to peanuts. In order to avoid a life-threatening reaction, I must avoid eating all foods that might contain peanuts, including:

artificial nuts
beer nuts
ground nuts
mandelonas
mixed nuts
monkey nuts
nut pieces
peanut
peanut butter
peanut flour
peanut oil

Please ensure any utensils and equipment used to prepare my meal, as well as prep surfaces, are thoroughly cleaned prior to use. Thanks for your cooperation.

Did you answer C? Peeling off the cheese and not eating that part of the bun won't ensure that you'll be safe. The protein (the part of the food that causes an allergy) in the cheese can contaminate the remainder of the burger and bun and cause a reaction.

6. The answer is B: Don't leave the house without your meds, no matter how much of a hurry you or your friends are in. Have the meds you need to treat a reaction with you at all times.

Did you answer A? Never assume that you won't need your meds. You never know when an accident will happen.

Did you answer C? If a reaction were to occur, symptoms could come on lightning fast, leaving you little or no time to get the proper meds. Additionally, certain meds your doctor may have prescribed aren't available over the counter, meaning you need a prescription for them. Don't be caught unprepared!

7. The answer is B: Pass on the bulk candy. There is a higher risk of accidental contact between foods in bulk bins, because some foods can get mixed in with others and scoops may be shared between bins.

Did you answer A? Skip the chocolate-covered raisins. Chocolate candy poses a higher risk for a reaction, as it is often manufactured on equipment shared with peanut-containing candy. Therefore, it is often recommended that individuals allergic to peanut avoid chocolate candy.

Did you answer C? Don't assume that your friend will know how to help you if you have a reaction. Taking a chance with a risky food just isn't worth it.

8. The answer is A: Bring your meds and store them properly. Temperatures can affect medicine. You should keep it out of the sun and away from extreme heat and cold.

Did you answer B? Medicine should never be left in a car, because you never know when you'll need it and you should therefore have it near you at all times. In addition, the inside of a car can get very warm. This can ruin the medicine and make it ineffective.

Did you answer C? By leaving your meds at home, you are taking a big risk. Accidents are never planned—carry your medicine with you at all times. It's better to be safe than sorry.

9. The answer is B: Practice what to do in the event of an allergic emergency. The troop leaders and your friends should all be made aware of your Food Allergy Action Plan.

Did you answer A? Never be without access to your meds. A cell phone, while helpful and a good thing to have access to in emergencies, isn't a substitute for medicine.

Did you answer C? Packing your own food is always a good idea, but keep in mind that even if you aren't going to eat anything else, you still need to be prepared to handle a reaction.

10. The answer is B: Calmly talk to your parents and tell them your side of the story. Work towards an open and honest relationship with them.

Did you answer A? By not telling your parents about the reaction and refusing to talk about it, you may lead them to question your responsibility.

Did you answer C? Yelling won't solve anything. Give your parents a chance to explain why they are upset. Pay attention to what they are telling you, and put yourself in their shoes. Explain your side and be honest—if you are worried that they'll yell at you for not being more careful, or if you think it doesn't matter since you already successfully handled the reaction, say so.

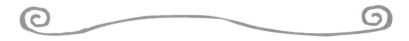

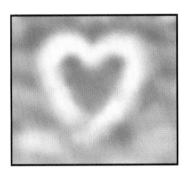

Share Your Stories

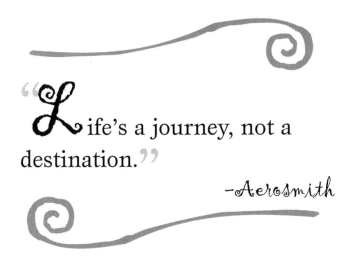

"Life's a journey, not a destination."

—Aerosmith

Share Your Stories

We hope that you have enjoyed reading this second volume of *Stories from the Heart: A Collection of Essays by Teens with Food Allergies* and that you realize that you are not alone.

As these stories show, almost everyone dealing with food allergies encounters similar situations and challenges. It is our hope that reading how others have handled such experiences and what they've learned from them, will help you with future situations you may find yourself in.

We also hope that reading these stories might inspire you to share one of your own stories with other teens with food allergies. Please send us any stories you would like us to consider for publication, or for posting onto our website, www.fanteen.org.

Send your stories to:

Food Allergy News for Teens
The Food Allergy & Anaphylaxis Network
10400 Eaton Place, Suite 107
Fairfax, VA 22030-2208
teens@fankids.org

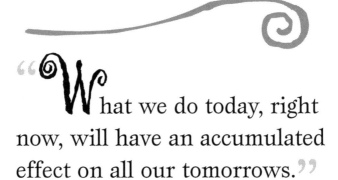

"What we do today, right now, will have an accumulated effect on all our tomorrows."

—Alexandra Stoddard

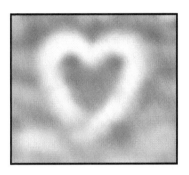

Other Sources of Information

"Never doubt that a small group of thoughtful, committed people can change the world, indeed it's the only thing that ever has."

–Margaret Mead

*T*he Food Allergy & Anaphylaxis Alliance is a group of international organizations working together to exchange information, form partnerships, and advance key issues of importance to those with food allergy and anaphylaxis.

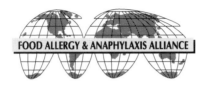

FOOD ALLERGY & ANAPHYLAXIS ALLIANCE

The members of the Alliance include:

The Food Allergy & Anaphylaxis Network
10400 Eaton Place, Suite 107
Fairfax, VA 22030-2208
Phone: (800) 929-4040
www.foodallergy.org
www.fanteen.org

Contact FAAN for educational materials about food allergy, including the booklet *Learning to Live with Food Allergies: Tips for Parents and Teens* and the videos *Food Allergy: Fact or Fiction!?!* and *Friends Helping Friends: Make It Your Goal!*. FAAN also hosts annual food allergy conferences with special sessions for teens, and publishes *Food Allergy News for Teens*, a free newsletter via e-mail. To subscribe, visit www.fanteen.org.

Allergy New Zealand
P.O. Box 56-117
Dominion Road
Auckland
New Zealand
Phone: 649 623 3912
www.allergy.org.nz

Allergy New Zealand works to improve quality of
life for people with allergies and their families
through support, education and information, and to
act as an advocate in all aspects of allergy.

The Anaphylaxis Campaign
PO Box 275
Farnborough
Hampshire GU14 6SX
United Kingdom
Phone: 01252 542029
www.anaphylaxis.org.uk

The Anaphylaxis Campaign provides a wide range
of fact sheets on food allergies, including a guidance
booklet targeted at teenagers. This booklet
specifically relates to nut allergy, which is common
in the U.K., but may also be helpful for teenagers
with other food allergies. The Campaign runs
awareness workshops for teenagers with allergies
around the U.K.

Anaphylaxis Canada
416 Moore Ave., Suite 306
Toronto, Ontario M4G 1C9
Canada
Phone: (866) 785-5660
www.anaphylaxis.ca

Anaphylaxis Canada offers cooking classes for
teens, an interactive teen website, and educational
materials. Contact this organization to find out
more.

**Food Anaphylactic Children Training & Support
Association (FACTS)**
21 Robinson Close
Hornsby Heights NSW
Australia 2077
Phone: 1300 728 000
www.allergyfacts.org.au

FACTS is a national, non profit, Australian charity
whose mission is to increase awareness about the
recognition and management of food allergy and
anaphylaxis, to provide education and support, and
to advance research on behalf of all those affected by
food allergy and anaphylaxis.

For support group information:

Support for Asthmatic Youth (SAY)
1080 Glen Cove Avenue
Glen Head, NY 11545
Phone: (516) 625-5735

This organization offers support groups for adolescents. Call or write to SAY to find out about a group near you.

For medical identification jewelry, contact:

Medic Alert Foundation
2323 Colorado Avenue
Turlock, CA 95382
Phone: (800) 432-5378
www.medicalert.org

To find a board-certified allergist, contact:

The American Academy of Allergy, Asthma & Immunology
Phone: (800) 822-ASMA
www.aaaai.org

The American College of Allergy, Asthma & Immunology
Phone: (800) 842-7777
www.allergy.mcg.edu

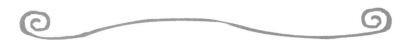